CLOSET
RESCUE

The Answer to the Age-old Cry
"I Have Nothing to Wear!"

JANISE FAITH
BACHLER
The Closet Diva

DEDICATION

To my Mom, who taught me about style because she was so stylish, and to my Dad, my rock, who always encouraged me to pursue my dreams and to stand on my own two feet. I am forever grateful for the sacrifices you made to provide me with a wonderful childhood and a good education.

To my daughters, Jessie and Gracie, who inspire me to be better at everything I do. I love watching you grow up and develop your own style. Your momma loves you and loves being your momma!

To my BFF, Catherine, for being my tireless cheerleader and always being there to me. You are precious to me beyond words.

To the rest of my loving family and amazing friends, who have loved and encouraged me on through all the challenges in my life in the past few years.

CONTENTS

ACKNOWLEDGMENTS

Thank you to Judith Rasband, founder and CEO of Conselle Institute of Image Management, who has been my teacher and mentor. Thank you to Ida-Jean (I.J.) McIntyre, and Patricia Morgan, of CAPS Calgary (Canadian Association of CAPS), and other CAPS members, for the great education you have provided and your encouragement in my speaking and writing career. Thank you to my editor, Lynn Stratton, from ClarityPro for your awesome suggestions and editing to make this book more readable for my readers. Thank you to my friend and printer, Rand Roeric, from Maranda Reprographics for your ongoing support (www.maranda.com). Thank you to Jana Miko from Miko Photography for making me feel and look beautiful in photos. Thank you to Britt Benjamin (www.brittben-jamin.com) for your wonderful artistic talents and the cartoons you created for my Closet Diva branding. And, thank you to my friend, Richard Heikkila-Sawan, for your ongoing patience and always making me look good with your amazing graphic design work (www.rhsimagine.ca).

1
INTRODUCTION

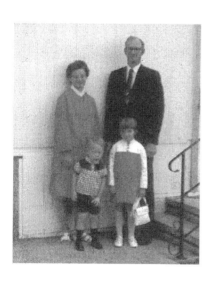
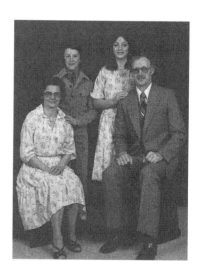

I have always loved clothes. My mom sewed clothes for me for years, including several mother/daughter dresses that still make me smile when I look at those pictures. My mom was incredibly stylish. I followed her around many a fabric store and pored over pattern books (anyone else remember Vogue or Simplicity?) picking out dresses for so many special occasions, including my graduation dress. I learned about fashion and

1

fabrics without even realizing I was learning. When I took my image consulting training in 2006, my teacher, Judith Rasband, was surprised by how much I knew about fabric. So was I!

I'll admit I went through some bleak times in my stylish life, like when I had each of my two daughters and ended up a bit on the frumpy side, carrying around extra pounds and being a stay-at-home mom, but thankfully, I always rebounded. By the time I was in my thirties, friends and family began to ask me to go shopping with them because "You always look great, Janise, and I don't know what to buy." This started my journey towards becoming a personal image consultant.

Then, in late 2005, I began to think it was time to leave behind the marketing and communications world I had been part of for 20+ years and try a new career path. I was considering home staging, because it was a new field at the time, but then our real estate market took a huge upswing and people were buying houses unseen, so that didn't seem like a good choice. It was also around this time TV shows began to feature makeovers, and I was in love with shows like "*What Not to Wear*" and "*Extreme Makeover*." So, in June 2006, barely a month after my now ex-husband announced that he didn't want to be married to me anymore, and with a very broken heart, I boarded a plane and headed down to Utah to take the image consulting training I had signed up for months earlier.

I am very grateful for both the distraction and the new focus my career in image consulting gave me as I struggled through the end of my 19-year marriage and re-invented my life with two young daughters in tow. It hasn't been an easy journey, but the journey is definitely easier when you are passionate about what you do. And I am passionate about helping women feel confident in how they look, because "*How you look affects the way you think, how you feel, how you act, and how others react or respond to you.*" (Judith Rasband, Conselle Institute of Image Management)

After you have worked through this "Closet Rescue" process, I hope that you can walk into your own, organized closet and be inspired to dress as who you really are. You'll walk out the door with your shoulders back, ready to take on the world, and become everything you were put on this planet to become.

I wish you all the best in your stylish journey!

Fashionably yours,
Janise Bachler, The Closet Diva

2 GETTING READY TO RESCUE YOUR CLOSET

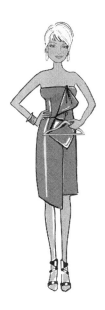

B efore a carpenter begins a project, whether it's a beautiful cabinet or an entire house, he gathers the tools that he will need. That's what your clothes are. They are "tools" to help you get what you want out of life. As Thomas Fuller once said, *"Good clothes open all doors."*

Of course, if the carpenter couldn't find his tools in the garage or his toolbox, then the tools wouldn't be very useful to him. So let me ask you, what state is your closet in? I am guessing, because you picked up this book, it's probably not great. Should someone put an "Enter at Your Own Risk" sign on your closet, like we sometimes do on the rooms of our teenagers? If so, this book is for you!

Our closets are often a much-neglected room in our homes. We don't take the time to organize and sort, because the task seems daunting. Closets tend to be small spaces, too, so just being in that space for any length of time can feel uncomfortable. But if you're thinking it's hopeless, it's not! I promise you that if you follow my "Closet Diva" process, which I do every week with my clients, you will soon be able to open your closet and find it a restful, blessed experience to walk into. You too can have a closet that inspires you, instead of stressing you out.

FIRST, GET READY MENTALLY

To begin this process, we need to get your mind ready. Before you pull one item out of your closet, I want you to sit down with a pad and pen and write out three to five reasons why you want to get your closet in order. This can be as simple as "So I can see what I have," or as complex as "I want a promotion and I need to dress better." Whatever your motivation, you will need to have some fairly compelling reasons, because if you don't, this process can be overwhelming. I am guessing you are already motivated if you purchased this book, but it is good to get clear about the "why." Once you have written your list, I want you to post it on the door of your closet so that you see it each time you open and close those doors during this process. This list will give you the "kick in the pants" you may need occasionally, because most people cannot do this all in one day.

SET ASIDE AN AFTERNOON

To start, I want you to set aside at least half a day. Some of you might need to take a day off from work or have a friend watch your kids for an afternoon so you can really focus on this process.

Although some of you who are the "Super Woman," Type A personality may be able to complete the process in one day, that will not be the norm. In fact, don't feel bad if it takes you several weeks. Just set aside a few hours a week, over the next few weeks, and you'll get the same results. But remember, no matter how long it takes, it will be worth it!

PREPPING FOR THE PROCESS

You will also need some very basic tools for this process:

1. **Notepad and pen** – This is for jotting down notes and "To Do" items for yourself, as well as any items you might want to put on your shopping list.

2. **Hangers** – I prefer to have hangers that match and are of relatively the same style and colour. Nothing looks messier than a mish-mash of plastic, wire and wood hangers. I especially dislike those wire hangers from the dry cleaner: They tangle easily and are hard on your clothes.

   I personally prefer white plastic hangers, some with non-slip grips on them, for jackets, tops and pants. You will also need some skirt hangers, the kind that squeeze the garment between two solid bars. Some people prefer wooden hangers, and while these are very nice, they take up a lot more space and are not very budget-friendly, especially if you are redoing your entire closet. I do, however, usually use wooden hangers when overhauling a man's closet, because they typically have fewer clothes and need them for dress pants and suit jackets.

3. **Rolling Rack** – This is an optional item but very useful if you have access to one, and you can use it later on to store off-season clothes (we'll talk more about this later). If you don't have access to a rolling rack, make sure your bed is made and available to hold clothes during your closet rescue.

4. **Boxes/Baskets** – These are also optional, but I find that some organizer-type containers are useful for items that look messy when they are simply folded on shelves, and they are also useful for holding socks or underwear.

5. **Specialty Racks** – In my own closet, I have a wall-mounted rack to hang my necklaces on, as well as a belt swivel, a scarf organizer, and a shoe organizer. These items can be purchased from most department stores, or you can find them on retail websites such as www.thecontainerstore.com or www.solutions-stores.ca.

AFTERNOON #1:

Now that you are ready to begin your closet rescue, I am going to share with you the rules we follow when I work with clients in their homes, and each rule begins with "Only have in your closet" …

Rule One: Items Related to Dressing

I have seen some interesting stuff in my clients' closets … novels, Christmas decorations, photo albums, sports equipment, baby paraphernalia (being stored for the next baby), and even a collection of vases. But your closet should not be a dumping ground or a storage room; when you open the doors, you want to feel the Zen, a feeling of tranquility and peace. You want everything before you to be about getting dressed, and you want to have everything you will need to do that.

One of my clients had several closets in her home, and she kept running from room to room, saying things like, "Oh, the shirt that goes with those pants is in my other closet." This is not productive. It wastes your time, and you will never know what you have when it is spread all over the house. The only exception would be outerwear: coats, shoes and boots, and winter scarves, gloves and hats. These can all be stored in a coat closet near the front or back door.

So, if you are using your master bedroom closet for storage, we want to remove all of that stuff and put it into another room. Do not attempt to put it away today, because we have more important things to do with your time than to decide where the Christmas ornaments should go. Just put the storage items in an adjacent room and move on. Ahhhhhh, now look at all the space you have, now that you've removed those items!

Rule Two: Items That Fit

Ladies, why do we have clothes in our closets that don't actually fit us? We have our fat clothes, our skinny clothes, and the clothes that actually fit. If you are anything like me, you could have two, three, or even four different sizes in your closet. Currently, I am size 8, so the only clothes in my closet are in that particular size. Why? Because I believe we already have enough guilt in our lives. Let me explain.

As women, we suffer from the "not good enough" syndrome in so many areas of our lives. We all experience guilt: We are not good enough mothers, or employees; we are not thin enough, or a "Suzy Homemaker," or the sex kitten we need to be in the bedroom. Trust me; there are few women who don't feel some guilt. We cannot do it all, and we cannot be it all. So why would we create more guilt for ourselves as we get dressed, knowing several (or quite a few!) items in the closet do not actually fit?

Let's decide today to be good to ourselves and take out every single item that does not fit us … right this minute! I don't care if you plan to lose 10 pounds this month. If it doesn't fit right now, it comes out. For those clothes we hope to get back into, I recommend you put them into a storage container, like a Rubbermaid tub, mark it "Size 8," or whatever size they are, and put them in the basement. If you actually do get down to that size again, then you can have a celebration when you bring up the storage bin and try on those clothes. I warn you, however, that the dress you wore to your high school graduation is probably NEVER going to fit you again, and it won't be in style anyway.

Now, for those "fat" clothes: I recommend you get rid of them completely. Do you really need a reason to gain weight? I don't. We already have enough temptation around us. Why give ourselves permission to gain weight because we have "back-up" clothes just in case?

Rule Three: Items in Season

This rule is one of the best things my mom ever taught me. As far back as I can remember, in spring and fall, as the weather was turning warmer or cooler, we would bring up the clothes from storage in the basement for the upcoming season and put our now off-season clothes into storage. It was a ritual I enjoyed with my mom, usually on the Easter and Thanksgiving long weekends, while we were out of school on holiday.

There are so many good reasons to do this. The first, and obvious, reason is that it frees up space in your closet; having off-season items clogging up your closet doesn't make sense. You aren't going to be wearing that wool sweater on a sweltering day in summer.

Second, it saves you time. If you are sorting through your clothes every morning, trying to find the right items for the season, it's a huge waste of your precious time.

But the third, and best, reason for removing off-season clothes from your closet is that it gives you a visual break from your clothes. This means you will not get as sick of them as quickly. It also means you will save money, because when you're not tired of seeing your clothes, you won't feel the need to replace them. When you bring up

Your closet should not be a dumping ground or a storage room; when you open the doors, you want to feel the Zen, a feeling of tranquility and peace.

10

your clothes for the next season, it is like having a whole new wardrobe. I promise you that you will forget what you have when you don't see it on a daily basis. You will be amazed at how excited you will be to wear the "new" clothes when you don't see them day after day, hanging in your closet!

You can store your off-season clothes in storage containers in your basement, or in a closet that isn't being fully used, such as one in a guest bedroom. I store mine in both. I have several Rubbermaid containers marked "Off-Season Clothes" (and "Off-Season Shoes") and I store them in my basement storage room. These are good for sweaters, jeans, shorts, T-shirts and other items that can easily be folded. My dressier clothes I hang in my youngest daughter's closet, which she hardly uses for her handful of dresses, her housecoat and a few hoodies. The rest of her closet is filled with my off-season clothes, my "fancy" dresses that I don't wear too often, and the home décor items and linens I am not currently using. I also change out my home décor colors and items seasonally. (I know, I know … I have some kind of strange sickness.)

Rule Four: Items in Style

If you are saving items of clothing because they might come back in style, I hate to be the bearer of bad news: Designers are not dummies. They don't want you to recycle your old clothes. They want you to buy the new ones. So they may bring back the essence of a trend, but it will be in a different way. That original trend will never come back in the same way, so unless it is a classic (more on this later), it is time to say good-bye to some of those items that are clogging up your closet.

If you are not sure whether something is in style, don't hesitate to ask your teenage daughter or a niece for their opinion. If they roll their eyes, chances are it is time to let it go. Or you could take the item to a local consignment shop. If the owner falls on the floor laughing over the acid-wash jeans you are trying to consign, it might be another clue that the style has left the building.

For those of you who have "memorabilia" clothing items hanging in your closet, like your wedding dress, or the dress you wore to your daughter's wedding ten years or ten pounds ago, I recommend boxing up those items, too. Mark them "Memorabilia" and put them in your storage room. Then you can decide next time you move if you really want to move them ... again. But for today, it makes no sense to take up valuable real estate in your closet if you can't wear them tomorrow. (Remember the romantic comedy, "27 Dresses," where ugly bridesmaid dresses entirely filled up one of her closets?)

What do you do with the clothing and accessories you remove permanently from your closet? Some people take their clothes to consignment stores. I personally do not have the time or energy to do that; plus, you may feel bad receiving a fraction of the actual cost of the item, especially when the consignment dealer marks it down if it has been hanging too long in their inventory. I always feel better when I donate my giveaways to my local Goodwill or Salvation Army thrift store for the benefit of others perhaps less fortunate than me. There are also many charitable organizations that will pick up your bags of clothing from your home, if you don't have the time to drop them off. But please do not donate items that are not in good repair or are just worn out; use them for rags or painting clothes, or simply discard them. No one else will want T-shirts with armpit stains, pants with holes, or that pilled sweater either.

3 EDITING AND SORTING

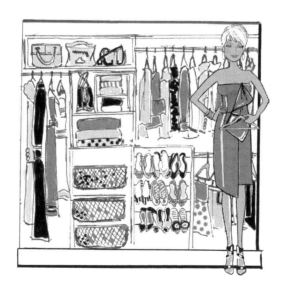

AFTERNOON #2:

Once you have removed all of the items that do not fit, are not related to dressing, are not in season, or are not in style, you should be standing in front of a closet that is filled with clothes that actually fit and are from the current season. It is far too overwhelming to do two seasons at once; I NEVER do it with my clients as a professional, so I don't recommend it for you as a "newbie" to the Closet Rescue process. Do your initial closet rescue with the current season only, and repeat this exercise when you bring up your clothes for the next season.

Step One: Remove all "home" clothes (the ones you would never wear out of the house!) and workout wear and put them on the bed. These do not usually need to be hung up, and they are best stored in drawers or folded on shelves after the Closet Rescue is completed. If you have outerwear jackets in your closet, remove them and hang them in a coat closet next to your front or back door, so you can get them as you are going out.

Step Two: Re-hang all clothes so they are facing the same direction, so that you can view them as you walk into the closet. You don't want to see the backs of the garments. This is a good time to switch over to using the same hangers, too. I also like to button one or two buttons on shirts, and one button on jackets, so you can see what they would look like on your body and they do not slip off the hangers.

Step Three: Hang every garment on a separate hanger. Do not hang suits together or have skirts doubled up on the same skirt hanger.

Step Four: Start from one end of the rod and sort all of your clothing by colour as best you can. Put all of the tops, bottoms and jackets/blazers together within colour categories. This is not how your closet will stay, but it is the way we get you ready to organize your closet in an exciting, brand-new way: into "clusters."

4 CLUSTERING

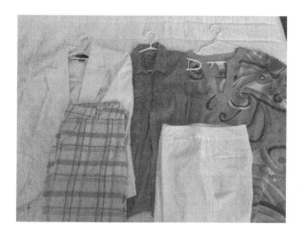

What I have seen in my work is that most people, if they have any type of organization in their closet, typically hang clothes in two ways: either by type (all pants together, all shirts together, and so on) or by colour (all blue together, all black together, and so on). Neither of these is conducive to getting dressed easily in the morning, although the colour system is definitely better than the type system.

I want to remove the stress in getting dressed for you, and I am going to do that by teaching you a revolutionary shopping and closet organizing system called "clustering."

A "cluster" is small group of clothing, typically 6-12 pieces, but it can be larger, based primarily on a function. A function is the type of cluster, or what it will be used for. Is it for work? Is it for the weekend? Is it for date nights? Is it for golf? Is it for vacation travel? Is it for work travel? Most of us will require several types of clusters in our wardrobe, and, depending on our lifestyle, we may have several clusters with the same function. For example, for someone who works full time, you may have two to three work clusters.

Secondly, a cluster is based on a colour theme. A colour theme is not based on one colour, such as black, but includes two to three colours, usually derived from a patterned piece that contains 2-3 colours. I call this piece an "inspiration" piece, because it inspires the cluster. This inspiration piece is typically a patterned garment, such as a blouse or top, a scarf, or even a patterned sweater or jacket. Fabric designers are brilliant at mixing colours; they understand the colour wheel much better than you or I, and so we need to trust them. An inspiration piece should contain 2-3 colours, with one of them a neutral.

Lastly, a cluster contains the components – bottoms, tops and layering pieces – to create outfits. A cluster should give you lots of mix and match options.

To explain this concept, let me start with an example of one of my own clusters, one I use for vacation travel to warm climates. My inspiration piece is a patterned silk tunic that contains pink, coral and white.

Using this inspiration piece, my first goal is to find three to four bottoms in my colour theme. For my cluster, I have the following bottoms:

Bottoms

- Coral drawstring linen pants
- White linen walking shorts
- Dark wash denim jeans
- Plaid, pink and coral walking shorts

You will note that I chose bottoms that are all different in size, shape, colour, texture, and even formality. You can also see that I have variety in my bottoms group, from casual to dressy, so that I can mix and match for various occasions.

Next, I selected four to six tops for my cluster:

Tops

- Patterned tunic (the "inspiration piece")
- Sleeveless, solid coral collared blouse
- White T-shirt
- Pink and white striped, ¾ sleeve T-shirt
- Pink shell (a dressier sleeveless tank top)

Lastly, and very importantly, I want to select two to three layering pieces. A layering piece is what makes an outfit! Too many women dress very one-dimensionally: They put on a top and a bottom and out the door they go. A layering piece (and/or accessories) makes an outfit. When you see someone who looks very "put together," it is usually because she or he has added a layering piece or smart accessories. Imagine a couch with no throw pillows on it: It is boring and sterile looking. The same goes for dressing. Your goal is to always put together an "outfit."

For my layering pieces, I selected:

Layering Pieces

- White blazer
- White cardigan
- Coral, long-sleeved linen shirt I can use as a "shirt jack" (shirt jacket)

There are some simple rules when purchasing or putting items into a cluster:

— *Each piece does not have to go with every piece in the cluster, but it should go with at least two to three other pieces in the cluster.*

For example, I probably wouldn't wear the patterned tunic with the plaid walking shorts, but both of those items go with almost everything else in the cluster.

When you see someone who looks very "put together," it is usually because she or he has added a layering piece or smart accessories.

— *Each piece should be different from each — no two pieces alike.*

I try to discourage clients from buying multiples of the same items. I once had a client who had four or five twinsets in her closet, but she really only wore one. The problem with buying multiples is that you wear the one that is in your favourite colour, and the rest go unworn. The one exception is if you want to purchase multiples in basics like white T-shirts or your favourite undies, but other than that, multiples are a no-no and usually a waste of hard-earned money.

I encourage you to find items for your cluster that are different in style, shape, color, line, texture, and even formality. This ensures that you will find it much more interesting to get dressed, and you won't get so easily bored with your wardrobe. Remember, our goal is to NOT have you standing in front of an over-stuffed closet, proclaiming, "I have nothing to wear!"

The very last step for your cluster is adding accessories. Start with basic accessories, like shoes or boots, and a great bag. Then gradually add in jewelry and scarves. I will talk more specifically about accessories in an upcoming chapter.

Keep in mind that you can continue to expand your cluster, or start a new one, when you need to refresh your wardrobe or have the desire to add a trendy piece to your wardrobe. I continue to add to my pink, coral and white cluster as I find pieces that work. And, sometimes, I retire pieces from a cluster because they are just plain worn out or the trend/style has come and gone.

Clusters are an excellent way to build a wardrobe, whether you are sorting your existing wardrobe into clusters or starting from scratch. Here are some excellent reasons why you would want to build your wardrobe using clusters:

1. **It gives you a plan.** Shopping with clusters in mind gives you a framework for how to buy clothes instead of shopping blindly. A lot of women find shopping overwhelming, and this is usually because they don't have a plan. Buying items to fit into an existing cluster or putting together a new cluster gives you a plan: You know what you are looking for, you know the colours and styles you are looking for, and you go out and find them!

2. **It saves you money** ... lots of money! Often, we wander around the mall hoping something will catch our eye. We pick up an item at one store that we like, and then another item at another store, and we go home. We might even spend a considerable amount of money on several items, but we get them home and they hang in our closets with the tags still on them because we have nothing to wear with them. What a shame!

3. **It eliminates orphans.** I go into my clients' closets all the time and find lots of orphans. What is an orphan? It is an item of clothing that doesn't fit into an outfit. It doesn't go with anything else ... except maybe jeans or black pants. We have already talked about dressing "one dimensionally," and this happens most frequently when we buy orphans. And then we wonder why we have a closet full of clothes and nothing to wear!

5 ORGANIZATION

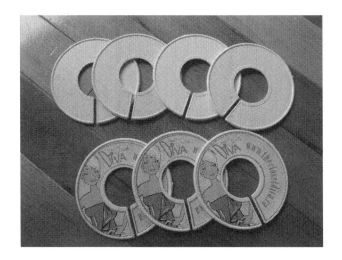

AFTERNOON #3:

Our goal for today is to hang all of your existing clothes in clusters. Why is this helpful?

- It helps you to dress more quickly because it makes the selection process easier.

- It helps you to see potential outfits.
- It helps you stay organized.
- It helps you to see "holes" in your clusters that you may need to go shopping for.

In our Afternoon #2, we sorted all of your clothes into colour categories, so this will make creating clusters a fairly easy task.

Choose one colour category to start with. We are now going to sort by type within each category, or cluster, by type and formality, as follows:

1. Take all layering pieces, such as jackets or blazers, cardigans, vests or V-neck sweaters, and hang them at the back of the colour category.

2. Next, take all of your tops and hang them in front of the layering pieces, with items with no collar first, then short-sleeved items, then long-sleeved items, and finally the collared items, which should now be right in front of your layering pieces. Collared items are more formal than un-collared items.

3. Lastly, hang all bottoms, with skirts first, then pants, capris and shorts. Skirts are more formal than pants, and pants are more formal than capris or shorts.

I use white plastic rings (which can be purchased at the Container Store), or closet rod dividers, to separate my clusters for myself and for my clients. And when you launder or dry-clean items, make sure you re-hang them within the cluster they came from. You can also write on those plastic rings which cluster it is, if that helps you visually separate the clusters.

Continue with the next colour grouping until you have sorted all of your clothing into type within each cluster.

Now pick one of your clusters and begin trying on different tops with pants and a layering piece, and see what kind of outfits you can create. If you have previously only worn the parts of one suit together, try wearing the skirt or pants with a different layering piece, like a cardigan or V-neck sweater.

Sometimes it helps to bring in a friend to give you their opinion on the outfits you are creating, or to give you some ideas. When you find an outfit you love that you haven't thought of before, write it down or take a picture of it that you can store on your smart phone or tablet for future reference when you have one of those mornings.

You will probably note that some of your clusters are pretty sparse. With your notepad or smart phone in hand, make a list of those pieces you are missing. Maybe you need more tops, or more bottoms? Maybe you need a shell to create another outfit? Maybe your closet is a sea of black

Clusters will take the stress out of getting dressed for your life.

(which I see quite often!) and you desperately need to add some coloured pieces? Or maybe your closet is a sea of solids and you need to add some pattern to your life? Make a note of the items you need to shop for in order to round out your clusters or to create more outfits.

NOTE: There will be some pieces within your wardrobe, such as jeans or khaki pants, for example, that can transition between clusters. That's OK. You can create a cluster of transitional pieces … or just hang them in the cluster where you think you will wear them the most, and take them out of that cluster for other outfits when you need them.

Now, you should be able to see a variety of outfits within each colour category, or cluster. When you get dressed in the morning, you can go from left to right, grabbing a bottom (usually based on the weather or the level of formality you need), a top and a layering piece and you are out the door! Talk about easy! Clusters will take the stress out of getting dressed for your life.

6 SHOPPING SMARTER

Before we ever step foot in a store, in order to address the "I have nothing to wear" issue, we must realize that we need to change our buying habits. We all know the old saying, "The definition of insanity is doing the same thing over and over again and expecting different results." If you really want to change the state of your closet, you cannot keep shopping in the same way. Here is what I recommend to my clients about changing their buying habits:

1. **Budget for Clothes** I recommend that you have a line item in your budget, just as we do for fuel or groceries, for clothing and personal care (haircuts, nails, and so on). Every month, if you put aside money for clothing, then you will have money to buy clusters instead of only one or two items. Trust me: it is a lot more fun to have several hundred dollars to go shopping with than being fearful of buying an outfit because your chequing account may not have enough in it to cover the cost. Remember, we want to buy outfits, and not orphans.

2. **Try on potential outfits!** If we want to buy outfits, we must try on outfits. During my shopping trips, I regularly see women taking one or two items into the change room, usually a couple of

tops. They seldom take any pants, layering pieces, or accessories to try on with those tops. When I take clients shopping, I will select enough pieces to create two different clusters. Usually, one colour cluster will be favoured over the other, and then we build on that favourite. I get my clients to try on 15 – 20 pieces at a time, with all kinds of "mix & match" potential; because my goal is to help my clients buy outfits, not orphans.

When you try on clothes, take in bottoms, tops, layering pieces, and even accessories, to create potential outfits. If the store policy allows only trying on a handful of items at a time, do not let this discourage you. Just ask the change room attendant to hold your other items to try on after you have tried on the first ones. If you don't take them all at once to the change room, I can pretty much guarantee that you won't go back out into the store and select more items to try on. Try to select six to twelve pieces to take in and try on together at one time.

3. **Spend money on classics.** It is wise to invest in clothing that will last, and these items are called classics for a reason. Classics have never been in style and never go out of style. Examples of classics are blazers, a pair of trouser dress pants, a trench coat, diamond stud earrings, a cashmere cardigan, basic button-down shirts, and boot-cut jeans. For classics like these, spend as much money as you can afford, because they will last you over many seasons. Spend less money on trendy items or trendy colours, because these will go out of style sooner. For a list of classics worth investing in, see the Appendix at the back of this book.

It is wise to invest in clothing that will last, and these items are called classics for a reason.

26

4. **Try not to "occasion" buy!** Many times we have the "I have nothing to wear!" moment when we need to attend a party, go out on a date, go to a job interview, or are invited to an event. We rush out to the store and buy something in a panic, which usually means we compromise and don't buy something that we love, but something that will do. When we do this, chances are we will never wear that piece or those pieces again. Try to anticipate these events and have potential outfits already waiting in your closet. If you have trouble remembering the outfits, take a picture of yourself wearing them and hang the photos inside your closet or put them into an outfit binder, or simply write down a description of the outfit for future reference. I take pictures and keep them on my iPhone and iPad for easy reference.

5. **Avoid the "SALES TRAP"!** If you fall in love with an item on sale, ask yourself this question: Do I have at least one or two things already at home in my closet that I could wear with this? If you don't, then ask yourself this question: Am I prepared, right now and today, to purchase two or three items to go with it to turn it into an outfit? If you have nothing at home to wear with it or you cannot afford to buy the other items to go with it, LEAVE IT ON THE RACK! Step away from the store! If you take it home, it will be just another orphan in your closet.

   Another good question to ask yourself about an item on sale is, Would I buy this if it was at regular price? If not, chances are you don't really love it as much as you should. I want you to be buying pieces that make you feel fabulous. I call them homeruns: If it isn't a homerun, don't take it home. If you get home and you are still thinking about that item a day or two later, then maybe you should go back and purchase it. It is always better to think about it and be sure than to "impulse-buy."

MAKING THE SHOPPING EXPERIENCE MORE ENJOYABLE

I encounter clients all the time who do not like shopping for clothes. This may sound unusual for a woman, but I assure you, it is not uncommon. Many women find walking into a store quite intimidating and even overwhelming. One of my clients even said to me, "Don't be surprised if I end up in tears." However, after teaching her how to shop smarter, she actually now enjoys the shopping experience and asks me to take her personal shopping almost every new season.

Here are a few pointers to reduce your stress when shopping:

- **Wear a nice but comfortable outfit.** You want to feel that you look nice, but today is not the day to wear your 4" stiletto heels, no matter how great they make you look. After an hour on hard tile floors, you will likely be in agony. (Oh yes, I have been there and done that!) Wear something that is easy to take off and put on. A button-up shirt or tights will be cumbersome and frustrating when trying on clothes.

- **Select your shopping venue.** If you find having too much selection overwhelming, avoid department stores and stick to smaller boutique or chain clothing stores in a mall.

- **Survey the merchandise for colour stories.** Stand at the front of the store and scan the selection before entering. In most chain clothing stores, at least the ones for grown-ups, you will see a number of colour groupings displayed. For example, on the right side, you may see clothing with various pieces in pink and black. Behind it you may see another group in coral and beige, and on the left, clothing featuring aqua and navy. In the clothing industry, we call these colour stories. Pick one or two colour stories, at the most, that appeal to you, and select four to six pieces from each colour story to try on. Why? The pieces within those colour stories are tonally dyed and selected to coordinate, for easier shopping for customers. This could be the beginning of a new cluster!

- **Ask for help.** Enlist the help of a salesperson immediately when you walk into the store. Most of us dread having a salesperson approach us asking, "May I help you?" Instead, intentionally choose a salesperson close to your own age, or one who seems friendly or knowledgeable with other customers, and get her on your side immediately. Just say, "I really need to put together one or two outfits today, and I could use your help." When the salesperson hears the word "outfit," she will usually be happy to help you because she knows you will be purchasing more merchandise than their average customer.

- **NOTE:** Keep in mind that salespeople are not trained image consultants. They are often underpaid and overworked, and their goal is to get merchandise out of the store, so when they tell you it looks great on you, be suspicious. Trust your own instincts and buy only what you love. Or, enlist the services of an image consultant or personal shopper who will give you her honest opinion, because the personal shopper's motivation is to make you look great so you will hire her again. A personal shopper does not usually make any commission off the sale of the clothing, so their motivation will be different than that of a salesperson.

Remember, above all, shopping should be fun. If you have some money in your wallet and a plan to buy outfits, or to add to an existing cluster, your shopping experience will be much less stressful for you, and you may even find yourself enjoying it.

7 SPICE IT UP WITH ACCESSORIES

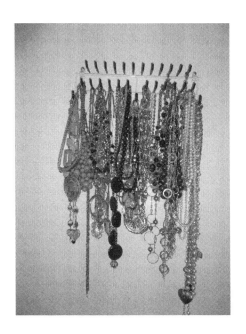

Accessories are to our wardrobes what spices are to cooking. As I said earlier, many women dress very one-dimensionally. Accessories help to create the layering that makes our outfits interesting and "spicy."

Handbags

I see so many women who miss out on a great opportunity to express their style and personality through the use of a great handbag, instead carrying a basic, utilitarian black bag that is often over-stuffed and worn out. What message does this kind of handbag send: "I am tired," or "I am boring"? Let's retire those black bags. Instead, find one in a fun colour or shape. You will be amazed at how many compliments you will get on it because you will stand out from the black-bag, utilitarian crowd!

Also, I recommend that you may wish to consider an "investment bag" if you have the budget for it. I used to buy a new handbag every season because, by the end of the season, it looked worn out and used up. My aver-

Let's retire those black bags. Instead, find one in a fun colour or shape. You'll be amazed at how many compliments you will get on it because you will stand out from the black-bag, utilitarian crowd!

age expenditure on a handbag was $40 - $50. Then, several years ago, my husband suggested we go look for a good bag for an anniversary present. I have to admit that I was intimidated just walking into the Coach store he took me to, but I tried on several bags and fell in love with a gorgeous grey patent leather "hobo style" bag. I seem to recall it cost $450.00! I almost fell over, but my husband insisted on buying it for me (gotta love that man!). I have used that purse almost non-stop for the past 4 years. I don't baby it. It has been on the floor of my car and many other floors, and to this day, it still looks brand new! I learned from this experience that you get definitely get what you pay for when it comes to handbags!

If you are going to buy an "investment" or name-brand bag, make sure you purchase a leather one. I don't love the cloth or faux leather ones; they typically look cheap, and the cloth ones get dirty and ratty in a hurry. Spend the extra money and buy a good quality bag in leather. The difference might be $100 or $200, but it will be well worth it in longevity.

Jewelry

I love costume jewelry! Having said that, I also like my fine jewelry. Aside from my wedding rings, I have several beautiful rings, necklaces and rings. A good way to get more mileage out of some of those smaller, finer pieces of jewelry is to layer them in with some costume pieces. This often has more impact and is more interesting than just wearing those pieces alone.

You may purchase costume jewelry specifically for a cluster that has the colours and style of that cluster; I do this quite frequently. When you do this, I recommend to clients that they take that jewelry and put it into a small, clear plastic bag, punch a hole in the top of it (just under the seal) and hang it on a hanger within the cluster. This way, you are never looking for that wayward earring in your jewelry case or the necklace that is all tangled up with another necklace.

How you store jewelry will also make a big difference in how often you wear it. If you can't locate your jewelry or it is too difficult to get out of the case, you probably won't wear it much. I worked with a client recently who had all her jewelry in their original little boxes in a storage container in her closet. I don't know how anyone can remember what they have when it is boxed up and put away. Here is how I recommend that jewelry be stored:

Jewelry You Wear Every Day:

You should dedicate a tray or container, or the top drawer of your jewelry box, for the jewelry you wear every day or quite regularly.

This tray might contain your wedding rings, your watch, a special necklace and so on.

Bracelets & Bangles:

I suggest a flat decorative box with compartments to keep on your dresser or in the bottom of one of your drawers for your bracelets and bangles. I also like the tiered jewelry organizers from the Container Store if you have room on the top of your dresser.

Miscellaneous Fine Jewelry:

You may wish to dedicate a drawer in your jewelry box for your fine jewelry, and you may also want to keep the necklaces in tiny plastic bags (the ones you get extra buttons in when you buy a new garment) so they do not get tangled.

Necklaces:

For those necklaces that aren't hung in with your clusters, you might purchase a jewelry rack with little prongs or hooks. If you place it on a wall in your closet, you will easily see your necklace selection, and it will keep them from tangling. If you want a great DYI project, find a wooden board or purchase a pre-finished one at a craft store, then purchase some smaller dresser drawer knobs (I love the selection at Anthropology because you can buy them individually). Simply screw them into the board at even distances. But if you're not a crafty person, you can purchase similar jewelry racks on Etsy (www.etsy.com) or at the Container Store (www.thecontainerstore.com).

There are many schools of thought on how to know how much jewelry to wear, but I have always gone by one simple rule: One piece of jewelry is the dominant piece, and the rest should be subordinate. In other words, one item is your focal point, and the rest shouldn't compete with it.

Keep in mind that when you layer several pieces together, the combination may create the impact of a dominant piece. For example, if you layer several necklaces together, that combination will become the focal point. If you then layer bangles on your wrist, that combination will compete with your layered necklaces, causing your overall look to become cluttered. A better plan is to wear a single bangle or a few thinner bangles together to simplify your look. I know of one image consultant who recommends that you accessorize your look, and then remove one item.

Watches are a "picky little detail" that can ruin your outfit. Studies have shown that men look at other men's watches to help them determine their financial status and net worth. Every man or woman should have a classy, all-metal or ceramic watch to wear with business attire. Watches with a leather band or funky coloured watches should be reserved for casual attire only. Wearing a cartoon character watch with a business suit may cause others to question your abilities, and your sanity.

Also, remember that your jewelry should match the formality and function of your outfit. You probably know that you shouldn't wear a sparkly pair of chandelier earrings with your golfing outfit, but I do see women who will wear them to work with their business attire. Remember the function you bought the earrings for? If the chandelier earrings were purchased to wear with an evening dress, chances are they are not appropriate to wear with a business suit. Dangly earrings can be quite distracting, so I caution you against wearing them for work. A simple hoop or diamond stud earrings are less distracting and a better option with your business attire. Leave the sparkly and dangly earrings for dates and other evening occasions.

When selecting your jewelry to accessorize your outfits, keep in mind the formality and function of your outfit. If you are wearing a hippie, "boho" type of outfit, then wooden beads and funky, colourful bangles will look great! But that same jewelry may not look so great with a dress for a formal occasion, such as a graduation or a wedding.

Jewelry, like your handbag, is a form of self-expression. Make sure you love every single piece you own. And remember that costume jewelry can get worn out and outdated, so you'll need to edit your collection occasionally.

Shoes

In my younger days, I chose vanity over comfort all the time. I was a size 7 and that was that. Now I no longer care about the number in shoes, just like I don't care about numbers in clothing. What is important to me is the fit. Yes, I still love a sexy shoe, but I buy it in a size 8 or 8.5, if necessary, to ensure that when my feet swell (and they always do!), I will not be in pain.

I think every woman needs several types of shoes in her wardrobe. Wearing the same pumps day in and day out to work not only gets boring, but the shoes will wear out faster. You need to alternate your shoes to make them last longer, so the leather or fabric has time to breathe and air out.

Here are the basic shoes I think every woman should have in her wardrobe:

Pump – Whether the toe is rounded or pointed, a mid-height heeled pump is useful for so many occasions. I think a black pump is the most practical, but it is nice to have pumps in tan, navy, and a couple of other fun colours for the summer months. Pumps are great with more conservative dresses, business attire, pencil skirts, dress pants, and even jeans.

Wedge – These are available in many forms, including cork, wood, espadrilles, and so on. Wedges are generally more casual and more comfortable, and they're fun to wear with a sundress or cropped pants.

Strappy Shoes – If you have a limited budget, a pair of strappy gold or silver shoes will serve you well for weddings and most formal events.

Flats – Flats or loafers are a good alternative to the ugly fitness runner for those marathon shopping trips, walking excursions, or commuting to work. I also carry a pair of thinner, fold-up flats in my bag when I am going out for the evening or when I am spending a long day in heels, so that I can slip them on to walk to my car, or when I just can't wear my heels one minute longer.

Boots – I think every woman should own one pair of dressier calf-high dress boots with a bit of a heel to wear with skirts, dresses and business attire. I also think a pair of casual brown or tan boots with a lower heel, or even no heel, are great with casual outfits.

Fitness Runners – These are great for working out at the gym or long walks, and these are the ONLY times that runners should be worn. There are so many other comfortable and more attractive options, like flats or sandals, to wear to the grocery store or for running errands.

NOTE: Having said all this, I am aware that some of you are limited to the kind of shoes you can wear because of various foot conditions. I want you to know that I sympathize with you. My mom has the same struggle. I wish I were the "foot fairy" but, alas, I am not. Although there are many specialty footwear stores out there, there are times when some women just cannot wear anything except the practical shoes designed to address their condition. In this case, just focus on, and play up, your best features, and no one will notice your shoes.

Outerwear

There are two mistakes I see women, and men, making when it comes to outerwear. The first mistake I see is wearing casual outerwear with business or dressy attire; there is nothing worse than seeing a man in a suit wearing his ski jacket to work. Every man and woman should own a classic wool or wool-blend outerwear coat in a neutral colour like black, navy, brown, tan or grey. A full-length coat will serve you the best, but you may also want to purchase a shorter, pea-length coat if you have the budget.

The second mistake I see with outwear is wearing a coat that is worn out or is in desperate need of dry cleaning, and lint all over your coat is not attractive, either. Coats generally wear out around the wrists and collar, or they just become so pilled that you can no longer even shave them. Coats need to be dry cleaned once or twice a season and replaced every two to three years.

Briefcases, Computer Bags & Totes

I once had a supervisor who carried his laptop and papers in a white-and-black backpack that needed a good laundering. I got so sick of it that when I left that job, I gave him a new laptop bag as a farewell gift. I could no longer stand to see him sending the wrong message to clients, because he was an accomplished man. Backpacks are for students, period. They are not for the grown-up world. With all the selections we have available to us, the briefcase, computer bag or tote that you carry to work or to meet clients does not have to be ugly. Many laptop bags are both beautiful and functional, so be sure to explore such wonderful options. They will complete your overall look every bit as much as other accessories will do.

8
PICKY LITTLE DETAILS

One small detail can ruin an outfit and in so doing can ruin the message you are trying to send through your appearance. This is unfortunate, but it doesn't have to be the case when you take care of the small details ... the "picky little details," as my teacher, Judith Rasband, referred to them.

Here is a list of "picky little details" that potentially could ruin your look:

- Too tight or too baggy
- Ragged, torn or soiled
- Snagged or pilled
- Wrinkled or rumpled
- Scuffed, dirty or unpolished shoes or boots
- Worn-out or dirty handbag or briefcase
- Using a backpack instead of an attractive tote or briefcase
- Outerwear coat that needs dry-cleaning or replacing
- Outerwear casual coat worn with dressy clothes
- Watch that is too casual

- Wearing "evening" jewelry or sparkle (such as sequins) to work
- Visible grow-out; roots need re-touching
- Dirty or chipped nails
- Rough heels or chipped pedicure (in summer)
- Too much perfume or aftershave
- Unshaven armpits/legs
- Armpit stains, spots or white marks

9 CREATING A DIVA CLOSET

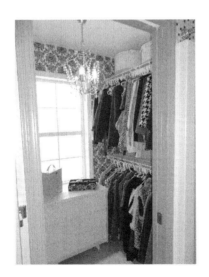

I don't know about you, but I often drool over pictures of huge walk-in closets that I see in magazines or online. These luxurious closets are larger than most of our bedrooms and outfitted with custom built-ins, beautiful flooring and lighting. We may not be able to afford a closet like that, but now that your closet is organized efficiently, you can turn getting dressed into a sumptuous experience.

CLOSET RESCUE

In my previous home, I had a very small walk-in closet, but I was fortunate to have a window in it. It had an inexpensive wire hanging system that I couldn't afford to replace, but here is what I did to turn my boring closet into a "Diva Closet":

- Had my dad help me wallpaper the back wall with gorgeous graphic, black and white wallpaper.
- Re-painted the other walls in a soft grey.
- Replaced the boring light fixture with a beautiful little chandelier I bought at IKEA.
- Purchased an inexpensive white furry throw rug to add some texture, and to cover the carpeting I didn't care for.
- Got an old dresser out of the storage room and painted it white for my underwear and socks, so I didn't have to leave the closet to get dressed.
- Purchased a new jewelry box with drawers and an attractive box with dividers for my bracelets, to set on top of the dresser.
- Purchased some round, decorative hat boxes to store my clutches and other handbags I wasn't using on a regular basis.
- Hung a floor-length mirror just outside the closet door for those last-minute checks.

I was very pleased with the results I saw from one weekend of work, and I believe it helped sell my home when I put it up for sale a few months later.

You may not wish to go to this extent, but you could use one or two of these ideas to give your closet personality ... your personality. Paint it a fun color or a soft comforting pastel, or simply buy a cheerful throw rug to put on the floor to brighten up your day. If you have the wall-space, in addition to your jewelry rack, hang a piece of artwork or a photo that inspires you.

Whatever you do to make your closet feel like a happy experience when you walk into it or throw open the doors, nothing will be more satisfying or more helpful to your life than having it organized.

10 AFTERWORD

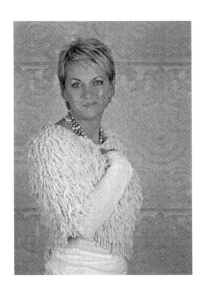

Alexandra Stoddard, one of my very favourite authors, in her book, "Living a Beautiful Life," says, *"I believe that if you take care of the small details, the big things take care of themselves. You can gain more control over your life by paying attention to the little things."*

Having a closet that is delightful to step into and is full of clothes you love, and is organized for the easiest selection, can help you do the big things you want to do.

I hope that the information in this book and my "Closet Diva" process will help you have fewer "I have nothing to wear" occasions. I am confident that by creating order in this area of your life, that you will have success in many other areas of your life. I wish you all the best in your journey.

Go forth and be glorious, my friends!

APPENDIX A

20 CLASSICS EVERY WOMAN SHOULD HAVE IN HER CLOSET:

- Trench Coat
- Wool coat for cooler months
- Jean jacket (fitted; not boxy)
- Tailored, one-button blazer
- Dark wash jeans (straight leg or boot cut)
- Khaki trouser pants
- Pencil or A-line skirt (knee-length; neutral colour)
- Straight-leg dark slacks
- Walking shorts or Capri pants for warmer months
- Cashmere cardigan
- Cashmere V-neck or scoop-neck sweater
- Tunic
- Crisp white button-down shirt
- Form-fitting T-shirt
- Cocktail dress (your favourite colour or the "little black dress")

CLOSET RESCUE

- Black pumps
- Strappy gold or silver heels
- Stylish flats or loafers
- Diamond stud earrings (real or cubic zirconia)
- Hoop earrings in gold or silver (small to medium)

ABOUT THE AUTHOR

Since 2006, Janise Bachler, the "CLOSET DIVA," has been helping men and women learn how to dress and to refine their personal image in a way that brings them personal and professional success.

Prior to opening her image consulting and speaking business, Janise spent 20+ years as a marketing and communications manager for both corporate and non-profit organizations before taking her image consultant training at the Conselle Institute of Image Management in Utah in 2006.

Janise has appeared on Calgary's Global TV & CityTV, has been interviewed on radio, featured in the Calgary Herald, and written several articles for local magazines. Janise has given presentations for such organizations as the Calgary Health Region, Mount Royal College, Red Deer College, Intuit Canada, Excel Homes, and many more.

If you want more great information on image management, as well as other resources and new books coming out, visit her website at www.theclosetdiva.ca. You can also follow her at Facebook/TheClosetDiva or Twitter @ClosetDiva_ca.

28114210R00033

Made in the USA
Charleston, SC
01 April 2014